Veterinary Antiparasitic Warfare

Strategies For Effective Parasite Control In Companion Animals

Genevieve Riversong Isabelle,Calloway

Table of Contents

1 **Introduction to Parasites** **5**
- 1.1 Parasite Biology 8
- 1.2 Lifecycle Stages 11

2 **Diagnosis & Identification** **15**
- 2.1 Microscopic Examination 17
- 2.2 Serological Tests 19
- 2.3 Molecular Diagnostics 22

3 **Endoparasite Control** **25**
- 3.1 Anthelmintics: Mechanisms 28
- 3.2 Anthelmintic Resistance 30
- 3.3 Treatment Protocols 33
- 3.4 Preventative Measures 36
- 3.5 Monitoring Efficacy 39

4 **Ectoparasite Management** **43**
- 4.1 Tick & Flea Control 45
- 4.2 Mite Infestations 48

5 **Integrated Pest Management** **51**
- 5.1 Environmental Control 53
- 5.2 Lifestyle Adjustments 55
- 5.3 Vaccination Strategies 58

6 Special Considerations **63**
6.1 Geriatric & Pediatric Cases 65
6.2 Pregnant Animals 68

7 Emerging Parasites & Threats **73**
7.1 Global Parasite Trends 75
7.2 New Drug Development 78
7.3 Research Directions 80
7.4 Zoonotic Implications 82
7.5 Future Challenges 85

1 Introduction to Parasites

Parasites, broadly defined, are organisms that live on or in a host and derive benefit from that relationship, often at the host's expense. Their survival depends intricately on their host; their life cycles are often incredibly complex, involving multiple stages and intermediate hosts. This intricate relationship dictates the strategies we employ for effective control. Understanding this fundamental interdependence is the cornerstone of successful veterinary antiparasitic warfare.

Many parasites exhibit remarkable adaptations to thrive within their hosts. Some have evolved sophisticated mechanisms to evade the host's immune system, while others manipulate the host's behavior to facilitate their own transmission. These adaptations, though impressive from a biological standpoint, highlight the constant evolutionary arms race between parasite and host, driving the need for continually evolving control strategies in veterinary practice. It's a complex interplay, a dynamic dance of survival. Failure to appreciate this complexity leads to ineffective treatments and potentially detrimental outcomes for the animal patient.

Consider the sheer diversity. We're not just talking about roundworms or fleas; we're encompassing a vast array of organisms, each with its unique biology and lifecycle. Protozoa, such as Giardia and Toxoplasma, are single-celled organisms with their own peculiar methods of infection and survival. Helminths, including tapeworms, roundworms, and hookworms, are multicellular creatures with often elaborate life cycles involving intermediate hosts like snails or insects. Understanding these differences is key to tailoring diagnostic and treatment approaches. A one-size-fits-all approach is doomed to fail.

Lifecycle stages represent critical junctures for intervention. Many parasites have specific stages where they are most vulnerable, whether it's during egg development, larval migration, or adult maturation. Targeting these vulnerable points offers the most effective approach to disrupting the parasitic life cycle and reducing infection. For example, many anthelmintics target adult worms, while preventative measures focus on interrupting transmission pathways. The precision required for successful intervention cannot be overstated.

Accurate identification of the parasite is pivotal for effective treatment. Microscopic examination of fecal samples remains a cornerstone of diagnosis for many internal parasites, allowing for the identification of parasite eggs or larvae. However, advancements in molecular diagnostics, such as PCR, provide greater sensitivity and specificity, enabling early detection of low-level infections and accurate species identification, even in cases where traditional methods may fall short. These modern techniques allow for more targeted therapy and help monitor the efficacy of treatment.

Furthermore, some parasitic infections manifest subtly, without overt clinical signs. Serological tests, which detect antibodies produced by the host in response to a parasitic infection, can be valuable in such scenarios, helping to diagnose infections that might otherwise go undetected. These tests are particularly useful in identifying chronic or latent infections where the parasite load might be low. Their inclusion in a comprehensive diagnostic strategy is crucial for successful outcomes. The selection of the most appropriate diagnostic tool, or combination of tools, depends on the suspected parasite, the clinical presentation, and the available resources. The holistic approach is paramount.

Beyond diagnosis, understanding the mechanisms of action of anthelmintic drugs is essential for effective treatment. Anthelmintics work through diverse mechanisms, targeting different aspects of the parasite's biology, from neuromuscular function to energy metabolism. However, the increasing prevalence of anthelmintic resistance necessitates a careful approach to drug selection and administration. This resistance, driven by the evolutionary pressures imposed by widespread drug use, requires a shift towards strategic and thoughtful implementation of anthelmintic therapy.

The prudent use of anthelmintics is paramount. Rotating anthelmintics, using combinations of drugs, and employing preventative measures are crucial strategies for delaying the onset and spread of resistance. Regular fecal examinations to monitor parasite burden and treatment efficacy are crucial elements of responsible parasite control. This responsible approach to parasite management is no longer a matter of convenience, but rather a necessity for maintaining the efficacy of currently available treatments.

Ultimately, effective parasite control necessitates a multifaceted strategy, encompassing not just drug treatment but also preventive measures such as maintaining good hygiene, controlling intermediate hosts, and implementing effective sanitation protocols. This integrated pest management approach is crucial in minimizing the burden of parasites on individual animals and the wider community. It's a holistic approach that views the parasite, the host, and the environment as interconnected components of a complex system. A balanced approach across several facets yields the best results. Effective parasite management requires an integrated and nuanced perspective.

Effective parasite control is not merely about combating existing infections; it's about preventing future ones. Strategies such as regular deworming programs, targeted environmental control measures, and the careful selection of environments where companion animals are allowed to roam all play a crucial role in minimizing exposure to parasites and preventing infestations before they take hold. Preventive measures are often more cost-effective and less invasive than treating established infections, offering a long-term solution rather than reactive interventions.

1.1 Parasite Biology

Parasites, by definition, are organisms that live on or in a host and derive benefit from it, often at the host's expense. Their survival hinges on a complex interplay with their host's immune system, environment, and their own intricate life cycles. Understanding this intricate relationship is fundamental to effective parasite control. The sheer diversity of parasites, encompassing protozoa, helminths, and arthropods, dictates the need for a nuanced approach to their management. Each species presents unique biological challenges requiring specific diagnostic and treatment strategies.

Successful parasitism relies on several key adaptations. Many parasites have developed sophisticated mechanisms to evade the host's immune system, masking their presence or actively suppressing immune responses. Others have evolved intricate life cycles involving multiple hosts or developmental stages, further complicating their eradication. For example, the complex lifecycle of the heartworm Dirofilaria immitis, involving mosquito vectors and various stages within the canine host, demands a multi-pronged approach to control. This includes preventative measures against mosquito bites, regular testing, and targeted treatment regimens.

Morphological characteristics often reflect a parasite's adaptation to its lifestyle and host. For instance, the flattened body of a tapeworm facilitates efficient nutrient absorption from the host's intestinal lumen, while the hooklets and suckers of some species enable firm attachment to the intestinal wall. Microscopic examination of fecal samples reveals these morphological traits, aiding in species identification. The specific structures, be they eggs, larvae, or adult parasites, are crucial for accurate diagnosis.

Understanding a parasite's physiology is equally vital. This encompasses their metabolism, nutrient acquisition, and reproduction. Many parasitic worms possess highly specialized digestive systems adapted to their specific environments within the host, be it the intestines or blood vessels. For example, blood-dwelling parasites have evolved intricate mechanisms for acquiring nutrients from the host's blood, often resulting in anemia. Knowing the metabolic pathways of a parasite can inform the development of drugs that target essential metabolic processes, thereby disrupting the parasite's survival.

Reproductive strategies are incredibly diverse among parasitic organisms. Some produce vast quantities of eggs, ensuring a high probability of successful transmission to a new host. Others exhibit complex sexual reproduction cycles, involving intermediate hosts for their larval stages. These diverse reproductive strategies influence the timing and intensity of parasite infections. For instance, seasonal variations in the prevalence of certain parasites often correlate with specific environmental conditions conducive to their development and transmission. Understanding these reproductive patterns is crucial for tailoring preventative measures and treatment timing.

The ecological niche of a parasite also greatly influences its life cycle and transmission dynamics. Environmental factors such as temperature, humidity, and the availability of intermediate hosts play crucial roles in parasite survival and spread. For example, certain ticks thrive in specific environments characterized by high humidity and vegetation suitable for their host animals. Understanding these environmental factors is essential for implementing effective control strategies.

In conclusion, effective parasite control necessitates a detailed understanding of parasite biology, encompassing their adaptations, physiology, reproductive strategies, and ecological influences. This knowledge forms the foundation for accurate diagnosis, the development of targeted therapeutic interventions, and the implementation of robust preventative measures. A holistic approach, considering the complex interactions between parasites, their hosts, and their environment, is paramount in achieving successful parasite control in companion animals. This detailed comprehension transcends simple identification; it's the key to informed decision-making in veterinary antiparasitic warfare.

1.2 Lifecycle Stages

Understanding the lifecycle of a parasite is paramount to effective control. Each stage presents a unique vulnerability, a specific point where intervention can be most effective. Neglecting this crucial aspect can lead to treatment failures and the perpetuation of infestations. A thorough grasp of these developmental phases allows for targeted and efficient strategies.

Many parasites exhibit complex lifecycles, often involving multiple hosts and environmental stages. Take, for instance, the heartworm Dirofilaria immitis. Its lifecycle begins with a mosquito vector, progresses through larval stages within the mosquito and the definitive canine host, culminating in the adult worms residing in the heart. Understanding each of these stages – from infective larvae to adult worms – is crucial for designing effective preventative and treatment approaches, such as preventative medication targeting the larval stages within the dog and controlling the mosquito population to break the transmission cycle.

Consider the intricacies of the Toxocara canis lifecycle. The eggs, passed in the feces of infected dogs, can remain viable in the environment for extended periods. These eggs then can be ingested by another dog, leading to a transplacental route where the larvae can migrate to various tissues. This highlights the need for meticulous sanitation and environmental control in addition to targeted anthelmintic treatments for both adult and larval stages. This highlights the importance of fecal examinations and the implementation of preventative measures. Failing to account for these varied stages would render treatment efforts ineffective.

The lifecycle of Giardia spp., a common intestinal flagellate, differs markedly. It involves the trophozoite stage, responsible for active infection within the gut, and the cyst stage, highly resistant to environmental stresses and easily transmitted through contaminated water or fecal-oral contact. Successfully managing giardiasis requires tackling both stages: addressing the active infection with appropriate medication and focusing on preventative measures such as environmental hygiene and providing clean drinking water. Interrupting the cyst stage's transmission is vital for effective control in affected populations. The persistence of the cyst stage further underscores the complexity of parasite control strategies, necessitating a multi-faceted approach.

The reproductive strategies of parasites also significantly influence their lifecycle dynamics. Some parasites employ asexual reproduction, leading to rapid population growth and increased transmission potential, exemplified by the prolific reproduction of certain fleas and ticks. Others utilize sexual reproduction, potentially leading to genetic diversity and increased resistance to control measures. Understanding these reproductive mechanisms is vital for designing effective control programs. For example, control strategies for fleas and ticks often incorporate environmental modifications in conjunction with animal treatments to target both reproductive and adult stages effectively.

Lastly, consider the impact of environmental factors on parasite lifecycles. Temperature, humidity, and rainfall influence parasite development, survival, and transmission. For example, the development rate of many parasitic nematodes is highly temperature-dependent. Therefore, environmental conditions must always be considered when developing parasite control strategies. Integrating knowledge of environmental influences into control programs is essential for enhancing their effectiveness and long-term sustainability. Climate change will likely alter parasite prevalence and distribution, adding another layer of complexity to parasite management. Climate change's potential to impact parasite lifecycles highlights the need for adaptable and comprehensive control strategies.

2 Diagnosis & Identification

Accurate diagnosis forms the cornerstone of successful parasite control. Without precise identification, treatment is essentially guesswork, potentially leading to ineffective therapy, prolonged suffering for the animal, and even the development of drug resistance. Therefore, mastering diagnostic techniques is paramount for any veterinary professional.

Microscopic examination remains a fundamental tool. Direct fecal examination, utilizing flotation or sedimentation techniques, allows for the visualization of parasite eggs, larvae, or even adult stages. This simple yet powerful technique provides immediate information on the presence and type of intestinal parasites. However, its accuracy relies heavily on the technician's skill and experience; misidentification is possible, particularly with morphologically similar species. Careful preparation of the sample and meticulous examination are therefore crucial. Beyond fecal samples, microscopic analysis of skin scrapings, blood smears, or tissue biopsies can aid in the diagnosis of ectoparasites and certain internal parasites respectively, enabling comprehensive diagnosis.

Serological tests offer a different approach, detecting antibodies produced by the host in response to parasitic infection. These tests, such as ELISA or immunofluorescence assays, are invaluable for identifying the presence of parasites that are difficult to detect through direct examination of samples or in cases of low-intensity infestations where parasitic load may be too low for microscopic detection. Serology provides a broader picture, indicating past or present exposure, but may not always reflect the current level of infestation precisely. It's also important to consider the potential for cross-reactivity with other related species, leading to false-positive results; this limits their specificity in some cases.

Molecular diagnostics represent a significant advancement. Techniques like polymerase chain reaction (PCR) offer unparalleled sensitivity and specificity. PCR amplifies specific DNA or RNA sequences from the parasite, enabling accurate species identification and even quantification of parasitic load. This high level of precision is particularly useful in cases of mixed infections or when dealing with cryptic or difficult-to-identify species. Molecular tests can also identify drug resistance genes, directly informing treatment choices and allowing for proactive management strategies. While PCR offers a highly specific and sensitive option, the technology requires specialized equipment and expertise, potentially limiting its accessibility in some clinical settings. Its cost may also be a prohibiting factor in many situations.

Integrating these various diagnostic techniques – microscopic examination, serological tests, and molecular diagnostics – is crucial for achieving a comprehensive and accurate diagnosis. The choice of test(s) should be guided by several factors: the suspected parasite, the clinical presentation of the animal, the available resources, and the cost-effectiveness. For example, a routine fecal examination may suffice for a suspected case of intestinal parasitism in a young, healthy animal. However, for a more complex case with atypical symptoms or suspected resistant parasites, more advanced molecular diagnostics may be necessary. A skilled veterinarian adept at utilizing a combination of these approaches ensures optimal diagnostic precision and aids in guiding effective treatment strategies. This systematic approach, incorporating multiple diagnostic tools as necessary, allows for better management of parasitic infestations in companion animals.

2.1 Microscopic Examination

Microscopic examination forms the cornerstone of diagnosing many parasitic infections in companion animals. It allows for the direct visualization of parasites or their diagnostic stages, providing crucial information for guiding treatment decisions. This technique, while seemingly straightforward, requires meticulous attention to detail and a thorough understanding of parasite morphology to ensure accurate identification. Proficiency in microscopic examination is therefore essential for any veterinarian working with companion animals.

The process begins with sample collection. Fecal samples, for example, should be collected fresh and examined as soon as possible to prevent the degradation of parasite eggs or larvae. Preservation techniques, like the formalin-ether sedimentation method, can be utilized for samples that cannot be examined immediately. However, it's crucial to remember that some preservation methods might affect the morphology of the parasites, potentially hindering identification. Careful and timely collection is therefore paramount.

Once the sample is obtained, a wet mount preparation is typically the first step. A small quantity of the sample is mixed with saline or Lugol's iodine solution, placed on a glass slide, and covered with a coverslip. Lugol's iodine, in particular, stains parasite structures, making them easier to see under the microscope. A careful scan of the slide at low magnification (10x) is then carried out to identify areas of interest containing potential parasitic elements, followed by higher magnification (40x and 100x) examination for detailed morphological assessment.

Accurate identification relies heavily on recognizing specific morphological features. For example, distinguishing between Toxocara cati and Toxocara canis eggs requires careful observation of their size and shell thickness. Similarly, identifying different species of Giardia cysts relies on the number and shape of the nuclei. Knowing these distinctions and practicing regular microscopic work will improve the accuracy of this important diagnostic process. Reference texts, illustrations, and even online resources prove essential in honing identification skills. This should be a standard part of your ongoing professional development.

Beyond fecal examination, microscopic techniques are applicable to various other sample types. Skin scrapings, for instance, are crucial for diagnosing mite infestations. Here, the choice of microscopy technique can also significantly impact the results. For example, while traditional light microscopy can reveal mites, dermatophytes, and other superficial parasites, more advanced techniques such as fluorescence microscopy might be necessary for detecting certain species or for a better visualization of specific structures. These advanced techniques may increase the diagnostic capabilities in certain situations.

Blood smears, too, can be examined microscopically to detect microfilariae, the larval stage of filarial nematodes. However, detecting these parasites can be challenging due to their low numbers and presence only in the peripheral blood at specific times. Therefore, techniques like Knott's concentration method are frequently used to enhance detection sensitivity, allowing for the visualization of these tiny creatures. This emphasizes the importance of knowing the life cycle of the parasites and selecting the most appropriate technique for each particular case.

Finally, tissue biopsies can provide valuable information about the presence and location of parasites. Examination of stained sections under a microscope allows for the identification of tissue-dwelling parasites, such as certain protozoa or larval stages of nematodes. The preparation and staining procedures are more complex than other methods and require more advanced skills. Yet the information obtained will certainly impact decisions regarding treatment and prognosis. Such procedures call for a deeper level of training and precise methodology. Learning to use these methods accurately will benefit your overall skills as a veterinary professional.

2.2 Serological Tests

Serological tests offer a valuable, albeit indirect, method for detecting parasitic infections in companion animals. Unlike direct methods like fecal examination, serological tests identify the host's immune response to a parasite, specifically detecting antibodies or antigens produced during infection. This approach proves particularly useful in cases where parasite detection through direct means is challenging, such as with low-intensity infections or when the parasite has a complex lifecycle, making direct identification difficult. The sensitivity and specificity of these tests, however, vary depending on the target parasite and the assay employed.

Several different serological techniques are available for veterinary use. Enzyme-linked immunosorbent assays (ELISAs) are widely used, offering a relatively simple, cost-effective, and high-throughput method for detecting parasite-specific antibodies. They are adaptable for use with various sample types, including serum, plasma, and even milk in some cases. Another commonly used approach involves indirect fluorescent antibody tests (IFATs), which visualize parasite antigens bound by antibodies in the patient sample. While IFATs often boast superior sensitivity, they require specialized equipment and expertise, increasing their cost and complexity compared to ELISAs. Western blot analysis provides another level of specificity, identifying individual parasite proteins involved in the immune response, which can help differentiate between various parasite species or even strains, proving valuable in scenarios with overlapping antigenicity.

The interpretation of serological test results requires careful consideration. A positive result indicates exposure to the target parasite, not necessarily an active infection. The presence of antibodies may represent a past infection, a latent infection, or even cross-reactivity with other related parasites. False-positive results can be observed due to various factors, such as cross-reactions with other pathogens or non-specific antibody binding. Similarly, false-negative results can occur, particularly during early stages of infection or in immunocompromised animals where the antibody response is suppressed. Therefore, veterinarians must always correlate serological test results with clinical findings and, whenever feasible, employ additional diagnostic techniques to confirm a diagnosis. This integrated approach ensures accuracy and guides effective treatment strategies.

Selecting the appropriate serological test is crucial for optimal diagnostic performance. Several factors need to be considered, including the target parasite, the prevalence of the infection in the local area, the sensitivity and specificity of various tests, and cost considerations. For instance, while ELISA may be a suitable choice for large-scale screening due to its high throughput, IFAT might be preferred in situations requiring high sensitivity, such as diagnosing low-intensity infections. Ultimately, the veterinarian's expertise and knowledge of available diagnostic tools are fundamental to accurate parasite diagnosis. The choice of test should always be guided by the clinical presentation, the epidemiological context, and the potential implications for patient management.

Beyond ELISA and IFAT, other serological approaches are increasingly explored within veterinary parasitology, constantly expanding the tools available. These include newer techniques like multiplex assays, allowing simultaneous detection of multiple parasite antigens within a single sample, increasing efficiency and cost-effectiveness for broader screenings. Additionally, ongoing research into specific parasite antigens improves the sensitivity and specificity of existing tests, enhancing their diagnostic capabilities. Furthermore, advancements in immuno-informatics are being used to develop more robust and accurate algorithms for analyzing complex serological data, leading to improved interpretation and decision making. As these advancements progress, veterinarians will have access to a growing array of highly sensitive and specific serological tests, allowing for ever-more precise diagnostics and optimized treatment plans. The future of serological testing in veterinary parasitology promises improvements in accuracy, cost-effectiveness, and ease of use, ultimately enhancing our ability to control parasitic infections effectively.

2.3 Molecular Diagnostics

Molecular diagnostics represent a significant advancement in veterinary parasitology, offering unparalleled accuracy and sensitivity in identifying and quantifying parasitic infections. Unlike traditional methods, molecular techniques, primarily polymerase chain reaction (PCR), allow for the detection of even minute amounts of parasite DNA or RNA in various samples, such as fecal matter, blood, or tissue biopsies. This increased sensitivity is particularly valuable in detecting low-intensity infections or identifying parasites present in low numbers, situations where traditional methods might fail. The speed and precision offered by PCR are game-changers in parasite diagnostics. Results are usually obtained within hours, drastically reducing diagnostic turnaround time compared to days or weeks needed for some conventional techniques. This rapid diagnosis allows veterinarians to initiate timely and appropriate treatment, maximizing therapeutic success and improving patient outcomes. Furthermore, molecular methods can distinguish between different parasite species or even strains, providing valuable information for targeted treatment strategies and epidemiological surveillance.

PCR's ability to detect even minute parasite DNA fragments is truly transformative. This enhanced sensitivity allows for early detection, before clinical symptoms manifest, enabling preventative interventions and minimizing the risk of severe disease progression. Imagine detecting heartworm infection early, preventing the devastating cardiovascular damage. Or detecting Giardia before it causes debilitating diarrhea. The ability to provide accurate, sensitive, and rapid diagnostics is an invaluable tool for improved patient care and public health. These techniques are also crucial for monitoring the efficacy of treatment, ensuring that chosen therapies are effective and preventing the spread of resistant parasite populations. By tracking parasite DNA levels over time, veterinarians can assess the effectiveness of treatment protocols and make adjustments accordingly, enhancing therapeutic efficacy.

The applications of molecular diagnostics extend beyond simple parasite identification. They offer the potential for accurate species-level identification, crucial when selecting appropriate anthelmintics or ectoparasiticides. Some parasites exhibit resistance to certain drugs, a knowledge molecular diagnostics helps provide. We can identify resistant strains and design treatment protocols accordingly. Molecular methods offer insights into the genetic makeup of parasites, giving researchers the opportunity to understand factors contributing to drug resistance, pathogenicity, and transmission dynamics. This understanding fuels the development of more effective control strategies and paves the way for innovative therapeutic approaches. Furthermore, molecular diagnostics facilitates epidemiological studies, allowing for the monitoring of parasite prevalence, distribution, and the emergence of new strains or species. This information is essential for public health measures aimed at reducing the spread of zoonotic parasites, those transmissible between animals and humans.

Beyond PCR, other molecular techniques are emerging and offer exciting new possibilities. For instance, next-generation sequencing (NGS) provides a comprehensive analysis of the entire parasite genome. NGS opens up avenues for detecting multiple parasite species simultaneously and even identifying novel parasitic infections. The level of detail that NGS provides on the parasite population dynamics, genetic diversity, and drug resistance profiles is unmatched by traditional diagnostics. This technology has great potential to revolutionize veterinary parasitology research, helping identify and address emerging parasitic threats. However, cost and specialized expertise remain challenges for widespread adoption of NGS. Microarrays and other high-throughput techniques, although also promising, have similar limitations.

However, widespread adoption of molecular diagnostics faces challenges. The cost of equipment and reagents can be substantial, potentially limiting accessibility for smaller veterinary practices. Moreover, specialized technical expertise is required to perform and interpret the tests, necessitating well-trained laboratory personnel or the use of commercial laboratories. While these constraints exist, the benefits far outweigh the limitations for many scenarios. Ongoing research and technological advancements are continually reducing costs and increasing ease of use. As these methods improve, the availability of rapid, sensitive, and specific molecular diagnostic tests will become more widespread in veterinary practice, substantially improving parasite control and animal health. Further, integrating molecular diagnostics into routine veterinary care will significantly enhance our ability to manage parasitic diseases in companion animals.

3 Endoparasite Control

The cornerstone of successful endoparasite control lies in a multi-pronged approach. It's not a one-size-fits-all solution; instead, it demands a comprehensive strategy tailored to the specific parasite, the host animal's age and health status, and the environmental context. Ignoring any one of these factors can lead to treatment failure and the potential development of resistance. This necessitates a nuanced understanding that goes beyond simply administering anthelmintics.

Effective treatment protocols begin with accurate diagnosis. Relying solely on clinical signs is insufficient; laboratory diagnostics are essential for precise identification of the parasite species and quantification of the parasitic load. This information dictates the choice of anthelmintic, dosage, and treatment duration. Microscopic fecal examination remains a fundamental tool, allowing for the detection of parasite eggs or larvae. More sophisticated techniques such as ELISA (enzyme-linked immunosorbent assay) or PCR (polymerase chain reaction) are invaluable in cases of low parasite burdens or when dealing with specific species identification challenges. These methods ensure that treatment is targeted and effective.

Anthelmintics, while crucial, are not a magical cure-all. Their effectiveness is contingent on several factors. Understanding the mechanism of action of each drug is paramount. Benzimidazoles, for instance, interfere with microtubule formation in parasitic cells; avermectins act on glutamate-gated chloride channels; and tetrahydropyrimidines inhibit energy production. This knowledge helps in selecting appropriate drugs and allows for informed decisions about treatment strategies for different parasite types.

Anthelmintic resistance is an escalating threat to effective parasite control. Overuse and improper use of anthelmintics have driven the evolution of resistant parasite strains, rendering previously effective treatments ineffective. This necessitates careful consideration of anthelmintic use; strategic drug rotation and the integration of non-pharmacological methods become crucial in the fight against resistance. Regular monitoring of treatment efficacy through fecal examinations is essential to detect the emergence of resistance, allowing for timely adjustments in treatment strategies. Avoiding blanket treatments of entire animal populations, and focusing only on those with proven infestation, can help to slow the development of drug resistance.

Preventive measures are just as important as treatment. Regular deworming programs, tailored to the specific parasite and risk factors, are vital in minimizing parasite burdens. This is particularly crucial in high-risk environments or with animals that have a high exposure risk. In addition to deworming schedules, proper hygiene plays a critical role. Prompt removal and disposal of feces, regular cleaning of animal living spaces, and controlled access to potential sources of infection can dramatically reduce the likelihood of infestation. These proactive measures lessen the reliance on anthelmintics, thus preserving their effectiveness and preventing the development of resistance. Implementing strong biosecurity protocols can also limit the spread of parasites between animals within a given environment, preventing outbreaks.

Beyond the core aspects of diagnosis and treatment, long-term success hinges on monitoring efficacy. Post-treatment fecal examinations are not merely a formality; they are an essential assessment tool. These tests provide critical information on the success of the treatment and the presence of any remaining parasites. If the treatment proves ineffective, a reassessment is required, possibly involving a change of anthelmintic, modification of dosage, or investigation into the potential presence of resistant parasite strains. Regular monitoring ensures that the chosen treatment strategy remains effective and allows for proactive adjustments to prevent treatment failure and the spread of resistant parasites. This continuous feedback loop is crucial to maintain long-term control.

The responsible application of these principles – accurate diagnostics, thoughtful anthelmintic selection, proactive preventative measures, and diligent monitoring – forms the foundation of comprehensive endoparasite control. It's a dynamic process that necessitates ongoing evaluation and adaptation to ensure the health and well-being of our companion animals. The ultimate goal isn't just to eliminate parasites; it's to implement sustainable strategies to prevent re-infestation and mitigate the broader implications of parasitic infections. This commitment to responsible parasite management safeguards not only the health of the individual animal but also the long-term viability of effective anthelmintic treatments for future generations.

3.1 Anthelmintics: Mechanisms

Many anthelmintics target specific parasite life stages, disrupting their metabolic processes or neuromuscular function. For instance, benzimidazoles like fenbendazole bind to tubulin, a protein crucial for microtubule formation, thereby interfering with parasite cell division and ultimately leading to their death. This precise mechanism explains their effectiveness against a wide range of nematodes. Understanding this specificity is key to effective treatment selection.

The macrocyclic lactones, such as ivermectin and moxidectin, exert their anthelmintic effects by binding to glutamate-gated chloride channels found in invertebrate nervous systems. This interaction increases chloride ion influx, hyperpolarizing nerve and muscle cells, leading to paralysis and death of the parasite. Importantly, this mechanism is selective, minimizing adverse effects on the mammalian host, a crucial safety aspect. However, individual parasite species show varying degrees of susceptibility.

Avermectins, a subclass of macrocyclic lactones, work in a similar way, targeting GABA receptors and glutamate-gated chloride channels. They disrupt nerve impulse transmission, resulting in paralysis and death of the parasite. However, the precise mechanism and efficacy can vary slightly depending on the specific avermectin used, for example, doramectin versus selamectin. These differences highlight the need for precise species identification before treatment.

The praziquantel family, commonly employed against cestodes and trematodes, acts on parasite cell membranes, increasing their permeability to calcium ions. This influx of calcium causes intense muscle contractions, disrupts tegumental integrity, and eventually leads to parasite death. Their effectiveness against flatworms is remarkably high, resulting in a significant reduction in parasite burden. It's important to note, however, these drugs don't affect all flatworm species with equal effectiveness.

Organophosphates, such as dichlorvos, act by inhibiting acetylcholinesterase, an enzyme essential for the breakdown of acetylcholine, a neurotransmitter. The resulting accumulation of acetylcholine leads to continuous stimulation of the parasite's muscles and nervous system, culminating in paralysis and death. This broad mechanism explains their efficacy against a variety of parasites; yet, these are often less favored due to higher toxicity concerns in companion animals compared to other anthelmintic classes.

Aminopentamidines, exemplified by pentamidine isethionate, display a different mechanism. These drugs interact with parasitic DNA and RNA, ultimately inhibiting their synthesis and replication. This effect directly targets parasite reproduction and growth, preventing the development of new generations. It's a promising mechanism, but its use is limited in veterinary medicine, primarily due to limitations in efficacy and safety profiles compared to other alternatives.

Niclosamide, frequently used against tapeworms, disrupts mitochondrial electron transport in parasites. This inhibits their ATP production, a crucial energy source, thereby compromising essential metabolic processes and ultimately leading to parasite demise. Its mode of action primarily targets energy metabolism, providing a different angle compared to drugs affecting neurotransmission or cell division.

Tetrahydropyrimidines, such as pyrantel pamoate and morantel tartrate, act as neuromuscular blocking agents. They selectively bind to nicotinic acetylcholine receptors in parasites, causing paralysis. The specificity of these drugs limits potential adverse effects in the host; however, the exact binding affinity differs between various parasite species, influencing their effectiveness. Clinical response varies accordingly. The effectiveness of anthelmintics hinges on factors like the parasite species, its life cycle stage, the drug's bioavailability, and the host's overall health. Therefore, accurate diagnosis is crucial for treatment success. Choosing the right drug based on a detailed understanding of these factors optimizes therapeutic outcomes and minimizes the risk of treatment failure or the development of resistance. Each anthelmintic discussed represents a unique approach in tackling internal parasites; a thoughtful selection, considering this specificity, is paramount. Precise identification of the parasite and an understanding of its life cycle remain crucial in selecting the optimal anthelmintic and treatment strategy.

3.2 Anthelmintic Resistance

The insidious creep of anthelmintic resistance poses a significant threat to effective parasite control in companion animals. It's no longer a hypothetical future; it's a current reality demanding immediate attention and strategic adaptation from veterinary professionals. The widespread use of anthelmintics, while initially highly effective, has inadvertently driven the selection and propagation of resistant parasite populations. This necessitates a paradigm shift, moving away from blanket treatments towards a more targeted, nuanced approach.

Understanding the mechanisms underlying anthelmintic resistance is crucial. Resistance can arise through various genetic mutations within the parasite, altering drug targets or enhancing drug efflux. Some parasites develop mechanisms that circumvent the drug's action entirely, rendering the treatment futile. Moreover, the development of resistance isn't confined to a single anthelmintic; cross-resistance frequently occurs, further complicating treatment strategies. Consequently, a single previously effective drug might prove wholly ineffective, leaving limited options for parasite control.

Strategic approaches to mitigate resistance are paramount. The cornerstone of this strategy involves judicious anthelmintic use. This necessitates moving away from routine, preventative treatments in healthy animals unless specifically indicated by parasitological examination or clinical signs. Instead, implementing targeted treatment based on rigorous diagnosis and species identification allows for the precise selection of an appropriate anthelmintic, reducing the selective pressure that fuels resistance development. This necessitates the proper use of diagnostic tools, as detailed in earlier chapters. Over-reliance on a single drug class must cease immediately.

Integrating diagnostic techniques into routine practice is essential. Fecal examinations, while crucial, aren't always sufficient for definitive diagnosis and identification of resistant strains. Sophisticated techniques like PCR and other molecular methods are often needed for accurate species identification and resistance genotyping. This allows veterinarians to tailor their treatment approach to each individual case, maximizing efficacy and minimizing the contribution to resistance development. This targeted approach is far more effective than blanket treatments, offering a greater chance of success in parasite control.

Developing effective treatment protocols requires a multi-pronged approach. Rotation or alternating anthelmintics from different drug classes can help delay resistance development. However, this requires a detailed understanding of cross-resistance patterns among different drug classes. Combining anthelmintics, though complex, can sometimes offer synergistic effects and provide a more powerful approach to parasite control. This strategy, however, requires careful consideration of potential drug interactions and potential adverse effects. Combining these treatments is not always safe and should be approached cautiously with careful monitoring.

Preventative measures remain crucial, but their implementation needs careful consideration in the context of resistance. Implementing stringent hygiene practices, such as regular cleaning and disinfection of animal housing, helps prevent parasite transmission and reduces the overall parasite burden. Similarly, controlling intermediate hosts, when applicable, can significantly reduce infection risk. However, relying solely on preventative measures without proper diagnostic surveillance can be a risky strategy, overlooking the rise of resistant strains.

Monitoring treatment efficacy is critical. This involves performing regular fecal examinations after treatment to assess the effectiveness of the chosen anthelmintic. A failure to observe a reduction in parasite load may indicate the presence of resistant strains. This underscores the need for subsequent diagnostic testing, including resistance genotyping, to guide treatment modifications. The effective monitoring of treatment efficacy necessitates that veterinarians continually re-evaluate treatment strategies based on the results, adapting the approach as needed to overcome resistance challenges.

Finally, fostering collaboration between veterinarians, researchers, and pharmaceutical companies is essential. Continued research into novel anthelmintic compounds is crucial to expanding our treatment arsenal. This includes investigating new drug targets and developing alternative parasite control methods. Furthermore, disseminating the latest research findings and best practices is critical to ensure all veterinary professionals are equipped with the knowledge and tools to combat the escalating challenge of anthelmintic resistance. Only through a collective, proactive effort can we hope to maintain effective parasite control in companion animals.

3.3 Treatment Protocols

Effective treatment hinges on accurate diagnosis. Once a parasite has been identified, the next crucial step is selecting the appropriate anthelmintic or ectoparasiticide. This choice must consider several factors: the specific parasite species, the animal's age, weight, and overall health, the severity of the infestation, and any potential drug interactions. Always consult the product label for dosage recommendations and adhere strictly to these guidelines. Overdosing can be harmful, while underdosing can lead to treatment failure and the potential development of drug resistance.

Many anthelmintics target specific stages of the parasite lifecycle. For example, some are effective against adult worms but not larvae, necessitating multiple treatments to break the life cycle completely. Others might be broad-spectrum, targeting multiple parasite species, making them ideal for cases of mixed infections. Knowing the target life stage is critical for successful treatment and minimizes the risk of repeated infestations. Careful consideration should be given to selecting an anthelmintic that is effective against the specific parasite species identified in the diagnostic phase of treatment.

Treatment duration varies depending on the parasite and the severity of the infestation. Some infections require a single dose, while others necessitate multiple treatments spread over weeks or even months. For instance, a heavy hookworm infestation might require a more extended treatment regimen than a light roundworm infection. Monitoring the animal's response to treatment is crucial. Regular fecal examinations post-treatment can confirm the efficacy of the chosen anthelmintic and guide any necessary adjustments to the treatment protocol. Always weigh the benefits against the potential risks, carefully evaluating potential side effects of medication.

The administration route also plays a significant role. Oral medications are most common, but some anthelmintics are available as injectables, topicals, or implants. Each route has advantages and disadvantages, and the veterinarian will choose the most appropriate method based on the specific situation. Injections, for example, can offer faster action and better absorption, particularly if there are issues with oral medication administration. However, they require more specialized handling.

Beyond simply administering medication, a holistic approach to parasite control is paramount. Effective treatment isn't solely reliant on pharmaceuticals. Consider environmental management – regular cleaning of animal living spaces, prompt removal of feces, and control of intermediate hosts (such as snails or slugs) where appropriate. These environmental modifications prevent the spread of parasites, minimizing future risks and the likelihood of re-infestation. Prophylactic measures like regular fecal examinations or preventative medications are equally important.

Always consider potential side effects. While rare, some anthelmintics can cause gastrointestinal upset, such as vomiting or diarrhea. Others may have more serious side effects, which are typically more significant in high-dose or repeated treatment settings. Before commencing treatment, carefully discuss potential side effects with the owner and provide clear instructions on what to monitor and when to seek veterinary attention immediately. Open communication is crucial, as early detection of adverse reactions can prevent severe complications.

For ectoparasites, a similar process of careful parasite identification guides treatment. Different insecticides target different parasites, and the choice depends on the species in question and any pre-existing conditions in the animal. This includes identifying ticks and fleas and treating based on this identification. Treatment choice will also depend on the severity and life cycle stage of the identified parasite. For example, topical treatments are easy to administer and often effective for fleas and ticks, while systemic medications may be needed for more extensive or resistant infestations. In cases of severe or extensive infestations, a combination approach, such as topical treatments supplemented with oral medications, may be beneficial. Always rotate treatment to avoid the development of resistance.

Regular monitoring remains essential. Even after apparent successful treatment, follow-up examinations are crucial. Parasites are cunning adversaries, and the development of resistance, undetected initial infestations, or environmental re-infestation are all reasons for regular check-ups and appropriate follow up treatment if needed. This monitoring enhances the chances of long-term parasite control and strengthens the protective protocols you have initiated.

The frequency of treatments will depend largely on the parasite life cycle, the efficacy of the treatment, the risk of reinfection, and the animal's overall health. Some parasites require regular treatment, whereas others might only require treatment periodically. For example, heartworm prevention is often administered monthly, while a single dose of broad-spectrum dewormers might suffice for a healthy adult animal in a low-risk environment. Regular discussions with the pet owner on preventative measures and their roles in minimizing parasite loads should be part of your consultation.

Finally, remember that treatment protocols must be tailored to each animal. Consider comorbidities and other medications the animal is receiving. This highlights the importance of a comprehensive history and thorough physical examination. Failing to account for these factors could lead to adverse reactions or treatment failure. Individualized treatment plans ensure successful parasite control without causing harm to the animal. Effective parasitic treatment is not a one-size-fits-all endeavor. Remember that responsible treatment includes thorough diagnostic testing, judicious selection of medications, careful administration, and consistent monitoring for both effectiveness and any adverse effects. Successful parasite control is an ongoing process, not a single event.

3.4 Preventative Measures

Regular fecal examinations are crucial. Think of it as a proactive health check-up, not just a reactive measure after symptoms appear. Early detection allows for prompt intervention, preventing parasite burdens from escalating into serious health problems. This is especially vital for young animals or those with compromised immune systems, where even minor infestations can have significant consequences. Regular vet visits, ideally every six months, should incorporate this crucial diagnostic tool. Don't wait for obvious signs; often, subtle changes in behavior or subtle clinical signs precede a full-blown infestation. Proactive monitoring is the key to successful parasite control. Remember, prevention is always far more effective, and far less expensive, than treatment.

Maintaining a clean environment is paramount. This involves regular cleaning of bedding, toys, and living spaces. Thorough removal of feces and any contaminated materials is essential. This simple act disrupts the parasite lifecycle, preventing the spread of eggs and larvae. For outdoor animals, regular grooming is incredibly important. This removes parasites, like ticks and fleas, directly from your pet's fur, reducing the chances of infestations. Consider using a flea comb regularly, especially in high-risk seasons. Remember, even seemingly minor parasites can create a considerable burden if left unchecked. Regular grooming significantly reduces this risk. A clean environment translates directly into a healthier, parasite-free companion.

Strategic use of preventative medications is vital, but should always be undertaken under veterinary guidance. There are various effective preventative medications available, targeted at different parasites. Your vet will advise on the most suitable product based on your pet's breed, age, lifestyle, and the prevalent parasites in your region. It's vital to follow the prescribed dosage and administration schedule carefully. Over\item or underdosing can impact efficacy or even cause health problems for your pet. Regular discussions with your vet are crucial; this ensures the medication remains effective and appropriate for your pet's needs. Never self-medicate; veterinary expertise guarantees the best and safest approach.

Careful consideration of your pet's lifestyle plays a significant role. For example, avoid walking your dog in areas known for high parasite prevalence, like heavily wooded areas or places with standing water. Regularly check your pet for parasites after walks or outdoor activities. Prompt identification allows for swift action, preventing the establishment of a significant infestation. Simple changes to your routine can significantly reduce your pet's exposure to parasites. This proactive approach can minimize the need for intensive treatment later on. This approach contributes to a healthier, happier life for your animal companion.

Dietary management can contribute to a stronger immune response. A balanced diet, rich in essential nutrients, supports your pet's overall health, enhancing its natural defenses against parasites. Consulting a veterinary nutritionist can provide personalized dietary recommendations tailored to your pet's specific needs. A robust immune system will naturally better resist parasite infestations, thereby reducing the need for extensive parasite control measures. Remember, a healthy diet is a foundation for good health, including parasite resistance. This supports the body's natural defense mechanisms and increases resilience to infection.

Effective communication with your veterinarian is crucial. Regular check-ups are more than just vaccinations; they're opportunities to discuss preventative measures, address concerns, and adjust strategies as needed. Open communication helps ensure your pet receives the best possible care, allowing for early identification of issues and prompt, effective treatment. Don't hesitate to contact your vet if you observe any changes in your pet's behavior or health, even if they seem minor. Proactive veterinary involvement optimizes parasite control and ensures the well-being of your companion.

Addressing the specific risks associated with your pet's environment is important. If you live in an area with a high tick population, for instance, regular tick checks and the use of appropriate tick preventative measures are essential. Similarly, if your pet frequently interacts with other animals, the risk of parasite transmission increases, requiring additional preventative steps. Tailoring your approach to your specific environment maximizes the effectiveness of your preventative strategies. A personalized approach ensures the effectiveness of any preventative measures. Your veterinarian can assist in identifying those tailored to your pet's specific circumstances.

3.5 Monitoring Efficacy

Monitoring treatment success is crucial; it's not just about administering medication, but ensuring it works. Failure to monitor can lead to prolonged suffering for the animal, ineffective treatment, and the spread of resistant parasites. Regular fecal examinations are the cornerstone of effective endoparasite monitoring, providing a direct assessment of parasite burdens. These should be performed before treatment to establish a baseline, then repeated at intervals specified by the chosen anthelmintic and parasite type. For example, a Giardia infection might require repeated testing within two weeks post-treatment, while a hookworm infestation might need monitoring a month later.

Microscopic analysis of fecal samples is the gold standard for many common intestinal parasites. Direct visualization of parasite eggs or larvae offers a definitive assessment of the treatment's efficacy. Quantifying parasite egg counts (EPG) provides a precise measurement of the reduction in parasite burden following treatment. A significant reduction in EPG indicates effective therapy, whilst a lack of reduction, or even an increase, signals treatment failure and necessitates reassessment of the treatment strategy. This may involve selecting a different anthelmintic, adjusting the dosage or frequency of administration, or considering alternative approaches. Remember that false negatives can occur; the best results involve consistently using the same microscopic technique to ensure comparability.

Beyond fecal analysis, other diagnostic methods can provide a more comprehensive assessment of treatment efficacy. Serological tests, measuring antibody levels against specific parasites, can indicate previous exposure and help track the success of treatment over time. However, serology alone might not be enough to definitively confirm elimination. More importantly, these serologic tests may not always be specific, leading to misinterpretations. For specific situations, advanced molecular diagnostic techniques, such as PCR, offer greater sensitivity and specificity for detecting parasite DNA. PCR can detect even low levels of parasitic DNA, providing a more nuanced view of treatment success, especially in cases where conventional methods might miss residual infections.

The choice of monitoring method depends heavily on the specific parasite, the chosen treatment, and the clinical context. For instance, monitoring for heartworm infection requires different approaches than monitoring for roundworms. It necessitates blood tests to detect circulating microfilariae or adult worms. In some instances, imaging techniques such as ultrasonography may offer insights into the presence and burden of internal parasites, particularly in situations where fecal examination proves unreliable. Thorough clinical examination, including assessment of the animal's overall health, weight, coat condition, and fecal consistency, also forms a part of the comprehensive monitoring approach. Improved appetite and reduced clinical signs indicate successful treatment. However, these general observations alone shouldn't replace laboratory testing.

Treatment efficacy monitoring isn't a one-time event. It's an ongoing process that's tailored to individual animals. Factors such as the animal's age, breed, concurrent health conditions, and the specific parasitic infection all influence the frequency and types of monitoring required. Regular monitoring not only helps evaluate treatment success but also plays a critical role in managing anthelmintic resistance. Early identification of treatment failures aids in preventing the emergence and spread of resistance. Moreover, timely intervention can prevent further parasitic damage, ensuring the animal's well-being and preventing the development of serious complications. Always remember to discuss the most appropriate monitoring plan with the owner to manage expectations and ensure compliance.

Consider the ethical implications of prolonged ineffective treatment. Continuing a treatment that isn't working causes the animal unnecessary stress and potential harm. It delays the implementation of appropriate strategies. Effective parasite management requires ongoing vigilance and a commitment to using the most current diagnostic and treatment techniques. Keeping abreast of research findings and advances in parasite control is crucial for staying at the cutting edge of effective parasite management. Remember that the veterinarian's expertise is vital in interpreting the results of monitoring tests and making informed decisions regarding treatment. A collaborative approach that involves regular communication with clients, ensuring their understanding and engagement in the monitoring process, ensures better long-term outcomes and fosters a strong veterinarian-client-patient relationship.

4 Ectoparasite Management

Effective ectoparasite management hinges on a multi-pronged approach, combining preventative measures with targeted treatments. Regular grooming, for instance, can significantly reduce flea and tick populations. This simple act not only removes parasites directly but also allows for early detection of infestations, enabling prompt intervention before they escalate. Thorough brushing, combing, and bathing with appropriate shampoos are crucial components of a comprehensive ectoparasite control strategy. Remember, consistent grooming isn't just about aesthetics; it's a proactive defense against these persistent pests.

Choosing the right treatment depends heavily on the specific ectoparasite. Fleas, for example, often respond well to topical insecticides containing fipronil or imidacloprid, applied monthly. However, always consult your veterinarian for dosage and application instructions, especially for small animals or those with pre-existing conditions. Misuse of insecticides can lead to adverse reactions, highlighting the need for professional guidance. Tick control, meanwhile, often requires different strategies, sometimes involving a combination of topical and oral treatments. The selection should consider the prevalence of tick-borne diseases in your region and your pet's individual risk factors.

For mite infestations, including ear mites, sarcoptic mange, and demodectic mange, diagnosis is critical. Microscopic examination of skin scrapings is essential for accurate identification. Treatment varies depending on the mite species. Sarcoptic mange, for example, necessitates systemic antiparasitics like ivermectin or selamectin, administered under veterinary supervision. Demodectic mange, characterized by hair loss and skin lesions, often requires a more prolonged treatment regime involving regular washes with medicated shampoos and sometimes systemic medications. Consistent monitoring of your pet's skin condition is essential to assess the effectiveness of the chosen treatment plan and to detect any potential complications.

Environmental control forms another crucial pillar of ectoparasite management. Regular cleaning of pet bedding, carpets, and upholstery can significantly reduce parasite populations and their eggs. Using appropriate cleaning products designed for parasite elimination further enhances this process. Treating the environment in conjunction with treating your pet ensures a more complete eradication of the infestation. Remember, parasites often complete their lifecycle within the pet's surroundings, emphasizing the importance of a coordinated approach that tackles both the host and its environment. Failing to address environmental factors can result in re-infestation, even after successfully treating the pet directly. Regular vacuuming and washing of pet areas significantly reduces environmental reservoirs of fleas and ticks.

Lastly, remember that effective ectoparasite management is an ongoing process, not a single-event treatment. Regular preventative measures, combined with vigilant monitoring, are essential for long-term protection. Scheduling regular veterinary checkups allows for timely detection of infestations and provides an opportunity for consultation regarding appropriate preventative strategies. In the case of re-infestation or failure of initial treatment, your veterinarian can tailor alternative approaches, considering factors such as drug resistance and your pet's overall health status. By establishing a proactive and comprehensive strategy, you can maintain your pet's health and wellbeing, shielding them from the significant discomfort and potential health risks associated with ectoparasites.

4.1 Tick & Flea Control

Effective tick and flea control hinges on a multi-pronged approach that integrates preventative measures with targeted treatments. Ignoring any component weakens the overall strategy, potentially leading to persistent infestations and associated health risks for the animal. The success of your chosen method depends heavily on understanding the parasite's life cycle and the animal's specific needs.

Regular grooming plays a surprisingly significant role. Thorough brushing not only removes existing ticks and fleas but also helps detect infestations early, allowing for prompt intervention before a large-scale problem develops. This simple, yet often overlooked, practice can dramatically reduce parasite numbers and transmission. Remember to carefully examine your pet's skin and coat after outdoor activities, paying close attention to areas like the ears, neck, and between the toes.

Choosing the right insecticide is critical. Many topical and systemic options exist, each with its own advantages and disadvantages. Topical treatments are convenient, offering localized protection, but their effectiveness varies with the product and the parasite. Systemic insecticides offer broader protection but require careful consideration of the animal's overall health and any potential drug interactions. Consulting your veterinarian to select the appropriate insecticide based on species, age, and health status is vital. Never administer medications without veterinary guidance. Improper use can lead to adverse reactions or treatment failure.

Environmental control is another cornerstone of effective tick and flea management. Regular cleaning of the animal's living space, including bedding and carpets, helps eliminate eggs and larvae. Using effective cleaning agents helps break the life cycle of these parasites. Consider using products specifically designed for parasite control and follow the manufacturer's instructions diligently to ensure safety and efficacy. Regular vacuuming is highly recommended, especially in areas where your pet spends the most time.

Beyond treatment and environmental management, lifestyle adjustments can further minimize exposure to ticks and fleas. Avoiding areas known to harbor these parasites is a simple preventative step. This includes avoiding tall grasses, overgrown vegetation, and areas frequented by wildlife. When engaging in outdoor activities in high-risk areas, consider using protective collars or other preventative measures. Regularly checking your pet for parasites after each outdoor activity is also essential.

While chemical control remains the mainstay of tick and flea management, exploring integrated pest management (IPM) strategies offers a more holistic and environmentally conscious approach. IPM emphasizes integrating multiple control methods – chemical, biological, and cultural – to minimize reliance on insecticides. This approach reduces the risk of insecticide resistance, improves long-term effectiveness, and contributes to environmental health. For instance, this might include using natural repellents alongside regular grooming and environmental cleaning. Consider the specific needs of your patient. Geriatric or pediatric animals may require modified treatment protocols due to age-related vulnerabilities or increased sensitivity to certain insecticides. Pregnant or lactating animals also necessitate cautious medication selection to ensure both maternal and fetal well-being. Always consult your veterinarian to develop individualized treatment plans. Never hesitate to seek professional veterinary advice when dealing with parasitic infestations. Early diagnosis and swift action maximize treatment success and minimize long-term health consequences. Accurate identification of the parasite is crucial in selecting the most effective treatment strategy.

The ongoing emergence of insecticide resistance necessitates ongoing vigilance. Regular monitoring of treatment effectiveness is essential. Regular veterinary checkups are critical in detecting new infestations or signs of resistance. This allows for timely adjustments to control strategies and prevents the development of resistant parasite populations. Stay informed about emerging trends in parasite control and new therapeutic options. The veterinary literature is a valuable resource.

Effective tick and flea control is a commitment, not a one-time event. Consistent application of preventative measures, careful selection of appropriate treatments, and regular monitoring will minimize infestations and promote your animal's overall health and well-being. Remember, successful parasite control requires a proactive and comprehensive approach, which begins with understanding the parasites' life cycles and adapting treatment strategies to the specific needs of the animal and its environment. A collaboration between owner and veterinarian remains crucial for achieving successful and sustainable control.

4.2 Mite Infestations

Mite infestations in companion animals present a significant challenge, demanding a multifaceted approach to effective management. Sarcoptic mange, caused by Sarcoptes scabiei, is a highly contagious condition characterized by intense pruritus, alopecia, and erythematous papules. Diagnosis often relies on skin scraping and microscopic examination to identify the characteristic mites. Treatment typically involves acaricides like selamectin, ivermectin, or amitraz, often requiring multiple applications to ensure complete parasite eradication. Environmental sanitation is crucial to prevent re-infestation, involving thorough cleaning and disinfection of bedding, kennels, and other areas where the animal spends time. The duration of treatment depends on the severity of the infestation and the animal's response to the chosen acaricide. Careful monitoring for clinical improvement is necessary, with adjustments to the treatment plan as needed. Ignoring environmental hygiene can easily lead to recurrent infestations and frustration for both pet and owner.

Demodectic mange, caused by Demodex mites, presents differently. These mites are usually commensals, only causing clinical disease in immunocompromised animals or under specific environmental pressures. Clinical signs can range from mild alopecia to severe, generalized demodicosis. Diagnosis relies on skin scraping and microscopic examination, focusing on the identification of the characteristic Demodex mites. Treatment options depend on the severity and extent of the infestation, ranging from topical therapies like lime sulfur dips for localized lesions, to systemic treatments like amitraz or milbemycin oxime for generalized disease. Immunosuppression plays a key role in demodectic mange, so addressing any underlying immune deficiency is vital for long-term control. It's also essential to consult with a veterinary dermatologist for severe cases, particularly generalized demodectic mange, as this often necessitates more intensive and specialized treatment protocols.

Cheyletiellosis, commonly known as "walking dandruff," is caused by Cheyletiella mites. It's characterized by intense scaling and pruritus, often accompanied by a noticeable dandruff-like debris. Direct visualization of the mites, which are relatively large and easily identifiable under a microscope, forms the basis of diagnosis. Treatment usually involves topical acaricides such as fipronil or selamectin, applied repeatedly until clinical resolution. Environmental control, similar to that employed in sarcoptic mange, is also essential to minimize the risk of re-infestation. The highly contagious nature of this infestation necessitates prompt treatment and preventative measures to safeguard other pets in the household or nearby environment from potential exposure. Failure to address the environmental components of the infestation can easily lead to prolonged clinical signs and difficulty in treatment.

Otodectic mange, caused by Otodectes cynotis, specifically targets the ears. This infestation presents with intense ear scratching, head shaking, and often a dark, waxy discharge. Otoscopic examination reveals the presence of the mites, which may be directly visible as small, white moving specks. Treatment typically involves topical administration of acaricides such as selamectin, ivermectin, or fipronil directly into the ear canal. Thorough cleaning of the ear canal is essential to remove debris and facilitate acaricide penetration. In severe cases, systemic administration of an acaricide might be considered, but topical treatments usually provide adequate parasite control. The severity of the infection can vary wildly based on the animal's general health and immune response, and neglecting early treatment can lead to chronic otitis externa.

Finally, always remember the importance of client education. Effective mite control requires a collaborative effort between veterinarian and owner. Detailed instructions on medication administration, environmental sanitation, and preventative measures are crucial. Regular follow-up examinations are necessary to monitor treatment efficacy and make necessary adjustments. Emphasize the importance of adherence to the treatment protocol, as premature cessation can lead to treatment failure and the development of acaricide resistance. Open communication and a thorough understanding of the mite life cycle and treatment strategy are essential for successful outcome and prevent relapse. Remember, patience and persistence are key elements in successful mite management, and the veterinarian's role extends beyond just providing medication to include comprehensive education and ongoing support for the client.

5 Integrated Pest Management

Environmental control forms the cornerstone of Integrated Pest Management (IPM). This isn't simply about tidying up; it's about strategically altering your companion animal's environment to minimize parasite exposure and breeding grounds. Regular cleaning of bedding, thorough vacuuming of carpets and upholstery, and frequent washing of pet toys and blankets directly reduces the parasite load. Consider the strategic use of insecticides in appropriate areas, always adhering to the label instructions meticulously, to further disrupt the parasite life cycle. For outdoor areas, managing vegetation and removing standing water, which serves as breeding grounds for many insects, can significantly reduce parasite populations. Remember, consistent and comprehensive environmental hygiene is key, preventing re-infestation after treatment. This approach also mitigates the risk of re-infestation, crucial for sustained parasite control.

Lifestyle adjustments are equally crucial components of a successful IPM strategy. Regular grooming isn't just about aesthetics; it's a proactive defense against parasites. Thorough brushing removes fleas, ticks, and their eggs, interrupting their reproductive cycle. Bathing your pet with appropriate shampoos, according to veterinary advice, can effectively eliminate many external parasites. Moreover, carefully monitor your pet's behavior. Unusual itching, excessive scratching, or changes in coat condition can all signal a parasitic infestation. Early detection, through diligent observation and preventative measures, allows for prompt intervention, minimizing the severity of the infestation. Be aware of potential exposure risk—avoiding parasite-infested areas like tall grass or areas with known rodent activity significantly reduces the chances of infestation.

Vaccination is not solely relevant to viral and bacterial illnesses; certain vaccines offer protection against parasitic infections. While not a replacement for other IPM strategies, vaccination can contribute to a multi-pronged approach that limits parasite burdens and transmission. Some vaccinations target specific parasitic diseases; their inclusion in a comprehensive wellness plan, following guidance from your veterinarian, should be discussed. For example, vaccines against certain types of heartworm are available and highly effective. The decision to vaccinate should be made on a case-by-case basis considering the individual animal's risk factors and lifestyle. These vaccines can reduce the severity of infections, minimizing the need for more extensive treatments and protecting against long-term complications. Consult your veterinarian for advice tailored to your pet's specific needs.

Integrated Pest Management isn't about eliminating every single parasite; it's about achieving a balance where parasite populations are maintained at levels that do not significantly impact your pet's health and well-being. This approach leverages multiple strategies, combining environmental control, lifestyle adjustments, and, where appropriate, vaccination. This holistic approach significantly decreases reliance on chemical treatments, minimizing potential risks associated with prolonged use or repeated applications. The goal is to build resilience in both your pet and the environment, thus creating a safer and healthier coexistence. Successful IPM demands careful observation, proactive interventions, and the ability to adapt strategies based on your pet's specific needs and your unique environmental circumstances. Remember that effective IPM relies on collaboration between you, your pet, and your veterinarian, fostering a long-term strategy for parasite control. It's a continual process that requires awareness, dedication, and careful management to ensure the ongoing health and well-being of your companion animal. Consistency is key to the success of IPM, with regular review and adjustments to the plan to ensure it's continually effective. Through this integrated approach you can minimize the impact of parasites on your pet's life.

5.1 Environmental Control

Maintaining a clean environment is crucial in preventing parasite infestations. Regular cleaning of pet bedding, food and water bowls, and living spaces dramatically reduces the parasite load. This simple act disrupts the parasite lifecycle, hindering their ability to reproduce and spread. Thorough vacuuming, paying particular attention to carpets and upholstery, removes parasite eggs and larvae. For hard surfaces, regular mopping with appropriate disinfectants helps further eliminate parasites and their residual waste products.

Proper waste disposal is equally vital. Prompt removal and disposal of fecal matter prevents the spread of parasites through the environment. This is especially important for areas frequented by pets, such as yards and gardens. Using sealed bags and depositing them in appropriate waste receptacles prevents contamination and reduces the risk of accidental exposure. Remember consistent practice in this area greatly limits the chance of reinfestation. For larger animals, regular cleaning of their living areas is essential. This can include cleaning out stalls, kennels, or runs, as appropriate.

Controlling insect populations is another critical aspect of environmental control. Fleas and ticks, for instance, often reside in yards, gardens, and even inside homes. Strategic use of insect control products, applied according to label instructions, is beneficial. This includes targeted applications in high-risk areas such as around pet bedding or entryways. Employing non-toxic alternatives wherever possible should be a priority, especially for household pets. Consider natural pest control methods such as introducing plants known for repelling insects into your garden or strategically using essential oils. It is extremely important to always carefully read and follow the instructions on any pesticide label.

Modifying the environment to deter parasite proliferation is equally important. Removing areas where parasites can thrive, such as excessive vegetation or standing water, limits their breeding grounds. Maintaining short grass and keeping the yard free of debris reduces parasite prevalence. Regular grooming of pets helps remove parasites and reduces the risk of infestation. This grooming regime, coupled with consistent environmental management, creates an effective defense against parasite incursion. This simple act drastically diminishes the chances of recurring infestations. Regular inspections of your pet's fur and skin can significantly contribute to detecting and mitigating infestations early on.

Beyond your immediate surroundings, consider the larger environment. If you frequently walk your dog in areas known for high parasite prevalence, consider switching to a different location. Regularly cleaning your pet's outdoor toys, such as balls or ropes, and keeping their food and water bowls clean when outside further reduces environmental parasite reservoirs. This overall approach significantly minimises environmental contamination and parasite exposure.

In conclusion, controlling the environment is paramount in preventing and managing parasitic infestations in companion animals. This approach involves a multifaceted strategy encompassing cleaning, waste disposal, pest control, environmental modification, and proactive measures to reduce parasite exposure. By adopting these strategies, you significantly reduce the risk of your pet contracting parasites and maintain a healthier environment for both you and your animal companion. The integration of these environmental strategies with other preventative measures, as detailed in other chapters, provides a comprehensive and effective approach to parasite control. Remember, a clean and well-maintained environment is the first line of defense in your veterinary antiparasitic warfare. Consistent attention to environmental factors plays a critical role in preventing parasite infestation and promoting the overall health and well-being of your beloved pet. Through diligent effort and a proactive approach, you create a safer and healthier environment for your pet, significantly reducing their exposure to and risk of contracting parasitic diseases. A well-executed plan focusing on environmental control provides a strong foundation for your overall parasite management strategy.

5.2 Lifestyle Adjustments

Regular grooming is paramount. This isn't just about aesthetics; it's a proactive defense against parasites. Thorough brushing removes loose hair, which can harbor fleas and ticks. Careful examination of your pet's skin during grooming allows for early detection of infestations, enabling prompt treatment and minimizing the spread of parasites. Consider the frequency of grooming based on your pet's coat type and lifestyle – a long-haired breed will require more frequent brushing than a short-haired one, and an outdoor dog may need more attention than an indoor cat. Remember, consistent grooming significantly reduces the parasite load.

Maintaining a clean environment is equally crucial. Parasites thrive in dirty conditions. Regular cleaning of your pet's bedding, toys, and living spaces is essential. Vacuuming thoroughly and frequently helps remove parasite eggs and larvae from carpets and upholstery. Wash bedding regularly in hot water to kill parasites. For outdoor areas, regularly remove feces and dispose of it properly, as many parasites use feces as a means of transmission. This proactive environmental management limits parasite populations, creating a less hospitable environment for their survival and reproduction. Don't underestimate the impact of simple hygiene on parasite control.

Dietary choices can unexpectedly impact parasite susceptibility. A balanced diet supports a robust immune system better equipped to fight off parasitic infections. Consult your veterinarian about the optimal diet for your companion animal, considering age, breed, activity level, and any specific health needs. Supplements, while not a replacement for preventative care, might, under veterinary guidance, boost immunity and overall health, potentially improving your pet's resistance to parasitic challenges. Remember, a healthy pet is better equipped to handle parasite infestations.

Careful selection of your pet's outdoor areas minimizes exposure to parasites. Avoid areas known to be heavily infested with ticks, fleas, or other parasites. Regularly check your pet for parasites after outdoor excursions, especially in high-risk areas like wooded trails, tall grass, or areas with standing water. Using preventative measures, such as topical or oral medications, before exposing your pet to high-risk environments can greatly reduce the risk of infestation. Educating yourself on the local parasite prevalence and taking preventative action are key steps in protecting your companion animal.

Understanding parasite life cycles helps you implement effective strategies. Knowledge about the specific parasites prevalent in your geographic region empowers you to tailor your preventative measures accordingly. For instance, understanding that heartworm is transmitted by mosquitoes helps you mitigate risk by using preventative medication and avoiding mosquito-prone areas during peak activity times. Learning about the specific life cycles of fleas and ticks allows for targeted interventions, like regular treatments and environmental control measures. Targeted interventions, based on understanding the parasitic life cycle, are crucial for effective control.

Social interactions influence parasite transmission. When your pet interacts with other animals, especially in areas with many other pets, the risk of parasite transmission increases. Limit contact with animals of unknown parasite status. If your pet participates in group activities like dog parks, be vigilant about checking for parasites after each interaction. Regularly consult your veterinarian about preventative measures and parasite testing, especially after interactions with other animals. Consider the risk factors inherent in social situations and act accordingly.

Regular veterinary check-ups are non-negotiable. Preventative care is the cornerstone of effective parasite control. Schedule regular check-ups with your veterinarian to discuss preventative medications, parasite testing, and any potential concerns. Your veterinarian can advise on the best course of action based on your pet's age, breed, lifestyle, and the prevalence of specific parasites in your area. Don't underestimate the importance of regular professional guidance in maintaining the health of your companion animal. This proactive approach dramatically reduces the risk and impact of parasitic infections.

5.3 Vaccination Strategies

Effective vaccination is a crucial, often overlooked, component of integrated parasite management. While anthelmintics and ectoparasiticide treatments target existing infestations, vaccines offer a proactive approach, preventing infection before it takes hold. This preventative strategy is particularly valuable in high-risk environments or for animals with compromised immune systems. Consider the significant reduction in disease burden and associated healthcare costs.

Several vaccines target key parasitic stages, disrupting their lifecycle and minimizing transmission. For instance, vaccines against Giardia spp. stimulate an immune response that reduces shedding of infectious cysts, thereby protecting both the vaccinated animal and the environment. Similarly, vaccines aimed at Toxoplasma gondii can lessen the severity of infection in susceptible animals, particularly those who might be vulnerable to the severe effects of toxoplasmosis. Remember that the efficacy of these vaccines, as with all vaccines, can vary depending on factors such as the strain of parasite, the individual animal's immune status and the administration techniques. Careful consideration of vaccination protocols is critical for optimal performance.

The selection of appropriate vaccines must align with the specific parasitic risks prevalent in a given geographic area and the animal's lifestyle. A dog frequently exposed to other canines in a park might benefit from a vaccine targeted against a common parasite prevalent in that setting, but a cat kept indoors likely faces different threats that require a targeted vaccine. Consult up-to-date parasite prevalence data for your region, consider the animal's age, overall health, and exposure factors. It's essential to note that vaccination alone rarely provides complete protection. Integrating vaccines into a broader parasite control program – incorporating preventative measures such as appropriate sanitation and regular anthelmintic treatment – is a far more effective strategy. Think of vaccination as one tool in a larger arsenal against parasites. A robust program employs multiple tactics for optimal results. This multi-pronged approach delivers a comprehensive solution capable of significantly reducing a pet's overall parasite burden.

Vaccination against parasites, like other vaccines, can generate mild reactions in some animals. These usually include minor localized swelling at the injection site or transient lethargy; however, serious adverse events are uncommon. Closely monitor your patients post-vaccination and be prepared to address any concerns. Open communication with pet owners about expected reactions and potential side effects is essential to build trust and ensure compliance with the vaccination program. Always have a plan in place should an adverse reaction happen. Record keeping, including documenting the type of vaccine, the date of administration, and any subsequent reactions, is vital for both animal care and epidemiological monitoring.

The successful implementation of vaccination strategies hinges on understanding several key factors, many of which need to be discussed with pet owners. Effective client communication will ensure that the vaccination strategy chosen will be effectively implemented. These include addressing any questions and concerns regarding vaccine safety, efficacy, and the overall cost-benefit analysis. It's important to establish a collaborative relationship, where clients are active participants in their pet's health management and a well-informed decision is reached by both veterinarian and client. Only in this way can vaccination strategies, and preventative parasite management, be more effective. Remember, client education empowers responsible pet ownership.

Cost-effectiveness is another vital consideration in vaccine selection. While vaccines can be a valuable investment in preventative healthcare, weighing their cost against potential treatment expenses for parasitic infections is important. This analysis should factor in the direct costs associated with the vaccine itself, administration, and any potential adverse effects. You may consider potential indirect costs associated with time off from work due to pet illness, expenses for treating complications and the risk of zoonotic transmission. A thorough cost-benefit analysis is essential for delivering responsible and economically feasible parasite control strategies.

Beyond the individual animal, vaccination programs contribute significantly to the broader public health. By reducing the prevalence of zoonotic parasites (those that can infect both animals and humans), vaccination protects not only pets but also their owners. This public health element is often overlooked, but is a crucial component in the overall impact of vaccination strategies. Remember, a healthier pet population is a healthier human population. The prevention of diseases and the reduction in the use of medications contribute to a healthier environment, and therefore to a reduction in the need for future treatment. This is vital to the sustainability of veterinary care itself, and underscores the importance of vaccination in preventative healthcare.

Finally, monitoring the effectiveness of vaccination strategies is paramount. Regular assessments of parasite prevalence in the animal population, coupled with post-vaccination monitoring of individual animals, will provide crucial data to inform improvements in vaccine protocols and strategies and help track changes in parasite prevalence in your area. This continuous evaluation and adaptation to emerging trends is essential in staying ahead of the ever-evolving challenge of parasite control in companion animals. Data tracking and reporting allows for the fine-tuning of strategies, thus delivering more effective preventative treatments. The data gathered is vital not only for your practice but for the wider veterinary community and to the development of better vaccines and parasite control techniques in the future.

6 Special Considerations

Geriatric and pediatric patients present unique challenges in antiparasitic treatment. Older animals often have compromised organ function, impacting drug metabolism and clearance. Reduced liver and kidney function necessitates careful dose adjustments or alternative medications to avoid toxicity. For example, aminoglycoside antibiotics should be used cautiously in geriatric animals with existing kidney issues, and dosages may need to be significantly reduced. Similarly, the use of certain anthelmintics, including those that have a high degree of potential toxicity in this demographic such as ivermectin, requires careful consideration and close monitoring for adverse effects. Monitoring kidney and liver function before, during and after treatment is essential to ensure patient safety and efficacy. Conversely, younger animals have different metabolic rates and developing organ systems, making them potentially more sensitive to certain drugs. Therefore, treatment protocols for puppies and kittens need to be adjusted accordingly, often involving lower dosages or specific formulations designed for smaller, immature animals. Pediatric patients may have a higher risk of adverse reactions, so regular veterinary monitoring is vital, especially with regards to neurological symptoms and gastrointestinal issues. The choice of anthelmintic will heavily depend on the specific parasite and the age of the animal, requiring a detailed understanding of pharmacokinetics in this vulnerable population. Careful consideration should always be given to the potential developmental effects certain drugs may have on growing animals.

Pregnant animals require a particularly cautious approach to parasite control. Many commonly used antiparasitic drugs, including several broad-spectrum anthelmintics, can pose a risk to the developing fetus. The potential teratogenic effects of these medications must be weighed against the risks of untreated parasitism to both the mother and offspring. Prioritizing the safety of the fetus necessitates a thorough risk-benefit assessment for each individual case, considering the stage of gestation and the specific parasite involved. The choice of drug should always be the safest and most effective while minimizing potential harm to the developing fetus. A detailed knowledge of the pharmacokinetics and pharmacodynamics of various anthelmintics in pregnant animals, including factors affecting drug distribution across the placental barrier, is crucial. In many instances, safer, less toxic alternatives might be available, possibly even requiring a change in treatment protocols. For instance, some natural products may be preferable, but only with the approval of a veterinarian. In some cases, preventative strategies, such as rigorous environmental control and diligent parasite monitoring during pregnancy, might suffice, while reserving more aggressive treatment only when absolutely necessary. It's imperative to consider the potential impact on lactation as well. Drug residues in maternal milk could potentially harm the newborn, making it vital to select medications with minimal lactational transfer. Thus, thorough communication and close monitoring are paramount, highlighting the importance of a personalized strategy for each pregnant animal.

The effective management of parasites in both geriatric and pregnant animals demands a nuanced understanding of their physiological vulnerabilities and the potential risks associated with various treatment strategies. Individualized treatment plans, tailored to the specific needs of each animal and the stage of their life cycle, are paramount for optimal outcomes. Regular monitoring for adverse effects and ensuring the proper drug dosage is crucial for the wellbeing of both the animal and its offspring. A collaborative approach between the veterinary professional and the owner is key to successful management, emphasizing the need for clear communication and a shared understanding of the treatment process and its potential implications. The importance of understanding the species of parasite involved and the potential risks both mother and offspring might face cannot be overstated. Choosing the right medication, considering the gestational period and the potential risks during nursing, requires a high degree of veterinary expertise and careful decision-making that protects both the animal and the future generation. Always prioritize the safety and wellbeing of the animal above all else, even when confronting treatment challenges. This careful approach is vital for responsible veterinary practice.

6.1 Geriatric & Pediatric Cases

Geriatric and pediatric companion animals present unique challenges in antiparasitic management. Their physiological differences compared to adults necessitate a tailored approach, prioritizing safety and efficacy while considering potential drug interactions and age-related organ function. For senior animals, reduced metabolic rate and compromised organ function, particularly liver and kidneys, necessitate lower dosages and potentially longer treatment durations of anthelmintics. Close monitoring for adverse effects, such as gastrointestinal upset or neurological signs, is crucial, and alternative, less toxic medications might be preferred. For instance, while a broad-spectrum anthelmintic might be effective in an adult dog, a gentler, more targeted treatment could be safer for a geriatric patient with underlying kidney disease. Regular bloodwork is advisable to monitor organ function during and after treatment.

The immature immune systems of puppies and kittens make them highly susceptible to parasitic infestations. A careful approach to deworming is vital, and frequently used medications like fenbendazole are considered safe for neonates, but always in accordance with the manufacturer's guidelines and veterinary assessment. The potential for drug accumulation and toxicity needs careful attention, and lower dosages or altered treatment schedules may be needed to prevent adverse effects. Moreover, preventing infestation is key. Strict hygiene protocols, controlling environmental parasites, and protecting young animals from exposure to infected feces are critical. Regular fecal examinations, beginning early in life, are essential for early detection and prompt treatment of infestations. Treatment decisions must consider not only the parasite's species and life cycle but also the animal's age and developmental stage.

Weight-based dosing is essential in both geriatric and pediatric patients. Incorrect dosing can lead to ineffective treatment in underdosing or dangerous toxicity in overdosing. Accurate weight measurement is crucial, using accurate scales rather than estimates. Always follow the manufacturer's instructions meticulously, and when in doubt, consult with a veterinary specialist for tailored guidance. The use of spot-on flea and tick treatments demands particular consideration. These formulations contain concentrated insecticides, and a smaller animal's surface area would be subject to a higher concentration of these products per unit area. Using appropriately labeled products for size and weight is essential, with careful consideration for the specific product's active ingredient and potentially required dilution.

Choosing the right antiparasitic drug requires careful consideration of the animal's age, specific parasite infection, overall health, and any pre-existing conditions. The potential for drug interactions with other medications the animal might be taking must be reviewed. For example, some anthelmintics can interact negatively with certain heart medications or steroids. A comprehensive history of the animal's medical profile is therefore critical in selecting the safest and most effective treatment, alongside regular follow-up monitoring. Specific consideration must also be given to the possible presence of comorbidities that might influence treatment decisions. For instance, a geriatric dog with a heart condition might have its treatment options limited to avoid further cardiac strain. Careful communication between the veterinarian and pet owner is paramount to ensure effective compliance with the treatment plan. This involves clearly explaining the treatment's rationale, dosage, duration, and potential side effects.

Finally, preventative measures are paramount. Regular fecal exams, appropriate environmental control (sanitation, regular cleaning, pest control), and lifestyle adjustments (limiting exposure to contaminated areas) play a vital role. The strategic use of preventative medications, like monthly heartworm preventatives, should be discussed and tailored to the individual's needs, considering both the age and health status. Remember, early detection and prompt intervention are always the best strategies for managing parasitic infections in geriatric and pediatric companion animals. Collaborating closely with a veterinarian throughout the process ensures a safe and effective treatment plan for your patients, leading to their improved health and well-being. A holistic approach, encompassing preventative measures, tailored treatment strategies, and vigilant monitoring, is critical for success.

6.2 Pregnant Animals

Pregnant animals present a unique challenge in parasite control. The primary concern is the potential harm to the developing fetus from anthelmintics or insecticides, necessitating a careful balancing act between maternal and fetal health. Many commonly used drugs are contraindicated during pregnancy due to potential teratogenic effects, meaning they can cause birth defects. This necessitates a thorough understanding of the specific drug's properties and the gestational stage of the pregnancy. Careful consideration of the parasite's life cycle is also critical; timing treatment to avoid crucial stages of fetal development is vital.

The selection of anthelmintic drugs during pregnancy must be highly specific. Broad-spectrum drugs, while effective against a wide range of parasites, often pose greater risks to the developing fetus due to their systemic effects. Narrow-spectrum drugs, targeting specific parasites, may be a safer alternative. Always consult comprehensive drug safety data sheets, paying close attention to the pregnancy safety categories established by regulatory bodies. This involves not only reviewing current literature, but also consulting veterinary pharmacologists and reproductive specialists for expert guidance when making such crucial decisions. This will minimize risks while effectively addressing parasitic infections.

The choice of administration route is just as significant as the choice of drug. Oral administration is often preferred, especially in early pregnancy to minimise direct fetal exposure. Injectable treatments, however, may be necessary in severe cases but demand greater caution and precise dosing. The potential for adverse reactions, including systemic toxicity, is increased. Precise measurements and calculations are crucial for minimizing risks, particularly when considering the physiological changes in the pregnant animal affecting drug metabolism and distribution. Careful monitoring of the mother's response to the treatment is crucial, paying close attention to subtle signs of toxicity.

In managing ectoparasites during pregnancy, the same principles of minimizing harm apply. Topical treatments, when appropriately formulated for pregnant animals, are generally preferred over systemic insecticides to reduce maternal absorption and minimize the risk of fetal exposure. However, effective control requires a thorough understanding of the targeted parasite life cycle. This dictates whether systemic treatment is really necessary, such as in the case of deeply burrowing ticks or other parasites requiring a systemic approach. Environmental control measures, including regular grooming and habitat modification, are essential adjuncts to the pharmacological management of parasites in pregnant animals.

Lifestyle modifications play a crucial supportive role. Careful monitoring of the animal's overall health, encompassing regular assessment of nutritional status, weight gain, and fetal development is paramount. Maintaining a healthy immune system enhances the animal's inherent ability to fight infection, lessening the need for extensive pharmacological intervention. A balanced diet, appropriate for the pregnant animal's nutritional requirements and the ongoing changes in her metabolic demands, is vital. This aspect helps support a robust immune response and supports overall health and wellbeing of the mother and fetus. A well-nourished animal is much better equipped to manage any parasitic burden.

Regular fecal examination is advised throughout pregnancy, to monitor the parasite burden and assess the efficacy of any treatment. The frequency of testing should depend on the risk factors of the animal's environment, the breed, and the prevalence of parasites in the region. This enables proactive interventions to prevent heavy infestations and minimizes the necessity for more intensive pharmaceutical interventions later on. Early detection and prompt intervention can help significantly reduce risk. Accurate identification of parasites is essential, guiding treatment choices and allowing for monitoring.

Preventative measures should commence well before pregnancy. Regular deworming programs, tailored to the animal's lifestyle and environmental exposure, can dramatically reduce the risk of heavy infections during pregnancy. Vaccinations, where available and appropriate, can also contribute to building maternal immunity against certain parasites and bolster the animal's natural defense systems. Careful management of the environment, minimising contact with potential sources of parasite infestation, is equally vital. These combined actions provide a multilayered approach to preventative parasite control.

The decision to treat parasites in a pregnant animal is not to be taken lightly. This requires weighing potential risks to the fetus against the potential harm of an untreated infection. Each case is unique and demands individualised assessment and management strategy. A collaborative approach, involving the owner, veterinary surgeon and other appropriate specialists, is crucial in making informed decisions, thereby providing the best possible outcome for both mother and unborn offspring. Open communication and a shared understanding are fundamental to success in this delicate situation.

7 Emerging Parasites & Threats

The rise of drug-resistant parasites poses a significant threat to companion animal health. We're seeing a concerning increase in the prevalence of previously rare or geographically restricted parasites, expanding their range due to factors like climate change, increased pet travel, and human encroachment on wildlife habitats. This necessitates a proactive and adaptable approach to parasite control, moving beyond the reliance on single-drug therapies. Developing integrated pest management strategies, that leverage a combination of preventative measures, targeted treatments and environmental modifications, becomes increasingly vital.

Effective parasite control relies heavily on accurate diagnosis, and this presents another challenge. Traditional diagnostic methods might not detect emerging parasites, or accurately differentiate between closely related species that may respond differently to treatment. This highlights the critical need for continued investment in and access to advanced diagnostic tools, including molecular techniques and sensitive serological assays. Furthermore, the ability to rapidly identify and characterize new parasites is paramount for timely intervention.

The development of novel anthelmintics and ectoparasiticides is crucial to counter the rising tide of resistance. This requires substantial research investment directed at understanding the mechanisms of drug resistance, identifying new drug targets within parasites, and exploring alternative therapeutic strategies, such as the development of parasite vaccines or immunotherapy. Collaboration between academia, pharmaceutical companies, and veterinary practitioners is crucial for efficient drug discovery and development. Ultimately, these novel treatments must be accessible and affordable to ensure their widespread use.

Globalization and increasing human-animal interactions significantly contribute to the spread of zoonotic parasites, those that can infect both animals and humans. Therefore, a One Health approach is essential. This means close collaboration between veterinary and human medicine professionals, public health authorities, and wildlife experts to monitor parasite transmission, develop effective control strategies, and implement public health interventions. Education of pet owners regarding potential zoonotic risks associated with parasites is also critical to minimizing public health concerns.

Predicting and mitigating future challenges requires sustained research efforts. This includes enhanced surveillance systems to track parasite distribution and prevalence, studies examining the impact of environmental factors on parasite populations, and research focusing on the development of parasite control strategies tailored to specific geographical regions and ecological contexts. A deeper understanding of parasite biology, host-parasite interactions, and the genetic basis of drug resistance will significantly improve the efficacy of parasite control programs in the long term. Investing in innovative technologies, like advanced imaging and data analysis, will help to monitor and manage evolving parasite threats more effectively. The future of companion animal health hinges on our collective ability to adapt, innovate, and collaborate to confront these ever-changing challenges.

7.1 Global Parasite Trends

The global distribution of parasites is shifting, a dynamic influenced by climate change, globalization, and evolving host-parasite interactions. Warmer temperatures expand the range of previously geographically restricted parasites, leading to increased incidence in regions previously unaffected. For instance, the northward expansion of tick species carrying Lyme disease is well documented, impacting companion animals and humans alike. This geographical redistribution poses considerable challenges for veterinary practice, requiring a reassessment of preventative strategies and treatment protocols. We're not merely dealing with a simple increase in parasite prevalence; we're facing a fundamental reshaping of parasite distribution patterns.

Globalization contributes significantly to the spread of parasites. The international pet trade facilitates the movement of infected animals across borders, introducing exotic parasites into new environments. These newly introduced parasites may lack natural enemies, allowing for rapid population growth and potentially significant health consequences for susceptible host populations. This underscores the importance of robust biosecurity measures at national and international levels. Failure to act decisively now will inevitably lead to substantial future challenges in terms of both public and animal health.

Furthermore, the complex interplay between parasite and host is constantly evolving. Parasites develop resistance mechanisms to existing anthelmintics and insecticides, rendering previously effective treatments ineffective. This necessitates a continuous search for novel therapeutic agents and integrated pest management strategies. The development of resistance is not merely a matter of individual parasite adaptation, but is often linked to genetic factors, the intensity of treatment, and the selective pressure exerted by agricultural and veterinary practices. The complex interplay between these factors requires a multi-faceted approach to combat resistance.

Moreover, climate change is exacerbating the problem. Altered precipitation patterns can influence parasite life cycles, increasing transmission rates and expanding their ecological niches. In certain regions, increased rainfall can lead to an expansion of mosquito breeding sites, increasing the risk of heartworm and other vector-borne diseases. Conversely, prolonged droughts can concentrate hosts and parasites, increasing transmission risks in localized areas. These complex interactions highlight the need for more sophisticated models predicting the impact of climate change on parasite distribution. Predictive modeling will help in proactive management strategies.

The emergence of new parasites and the resurgence of previously controlled infections are significant global trends. These trends, often linked to climate change and human activities, create urgent health challenges. Examples include the expanding geographical range of Leishmania, a protozoan parasite causing visceral leishmaniosis, and the increasing prevalence of drug-resistant ticks. These shifts demand a proactive approach, integrating advanced diagnostic techniques, novel treatment strategies, and effective public health interventions. These new parasites present a very dynamic and potentially dangerous scenario.

The consequences of these global trends extend beyond animal health. Many parasites have zoonotic potential, meaning they can be transmitted from animals to humans. This adds a public health dimension to parasite control, underscoring the need for One Health approaches that integrate veterinary, human, and environmental medicine. The emergence of novel parasites or the spread of existing parasites to new areas often carry severe implications for global public health, necessitating improved surveillance and prompt responses. An integrated approach becomes essential for effective disease prevention and control.

Effective strategies for mitigating these trends must be multi-faceted. They demand a comprehensive understanding of parasite biology, ecology, and transmission dynamics. This understanding is crucial for tailoring effective control measures, including the judicious use of anthelmintics and insecticides, implementing robust biosecurity measures, and incorporating integrated pest management strategies. Regular monitoring of parasite prevalence and resistance patterns is also essential to guide management decisions. Sustainable and effective parasite control requires both prevention and targeted intervention.

Finally, international collaboration and information sharing are paramount in addressing global parasite trends. The sharing of data on parasite distribution, resistance patterns, and novel treatment strategies facilitates the development of effective global strategies. Strengthening veterinary public health infrastructures in developing countries and raising awareness among pet owners about parasite prevention are also crucial steps. By working collaboratively, we can improve global health outcomes for both animals and humans. This collaborative endeavor is crucial for a successful global response to this serious threat.

7.2 New Drug Development

The relentless rise of anthelmintic resistance necessitates a concerted effort towards new drug development. Current treatments are losing their effectiveness, demanding innovative approaches to combat increasingly resilient parasite populations. We are facing a critical juncture where proactive measures are no longer optional, but essential for maintaining the health of our companion animals. The cost of inaction is far too high.

Focusing on novel mechanisms of action is crucial. Research should prioritize compounds targeting unique parasite metabolic pathways or essential biological processes not exploited by existing anthelmintics. This includes exploring natural products and repurposing existing drugs for veterinary applications. A multi-pronged approach, using both traditional pharmacology and cutting-edge technologies, is required.

One promising avenue lies in the development of drugs that specifically target parasite-specific proteins, receptors, or enzymes. This targeted approach minimizes off-target effects and reduces the likelihood of adverse reactions in the host animal. Sophisticated molecular modeling and high-throughput screening techniques allow for the efficient identification and evaluation of potential drug candidates. This rigorous screening process is vital to ensure safety and efficacy.

The development of combination therapies presents another powerful strategy. Combining anthelmintics with different mechanisms of action reduces the likelihood of resistance development. It also enhances therapeutic effectiveness, often leading to a lower dosage of individual drugs, thereby minimizing potential side effects. This synergistic approach offers a potent solution for tackling multi-drug resistant parasites.

Beyond traditional drug development, innovative drug delivery systems are pivotal. Targeted drug delivery systems can improve drug bioavailability, reduce systemic toxicity, and enhance the efficacy of anthelmintics. Nanoparticle-based drug delivery is a rapidly advancing field with the potential to revolutionize the treatment of parasitic infections. The controlled release of the drug directly at the target site significantly improves therapeutic efficacy while limiting exposure to other systems.

Collaborations between academic institutions, pharmaceutical companies, and veterinary practitioners are critical for accelerating the drug development process. Sharing research findings, streamlining regulatory processes, and facilitating access to funding are all essential aspects of collaborative efforts. Strong partnerships ensure the rapid translation of promising research into effective treatments. There is strength in numbers, and only through collaborative efforts will we meet the challenge.

Furthermore, a thorough understanding of the parasite's biology and its interactions with the host's immune system are crucial for the design of effective drugs. Understanding these details helps to identify potential vulnerabilities and facilitates the development of more targeted and potent therapies. This requires extensive research on parasite genetics, genomics, and proteomics to identify suitable drug targets. This deep dive into the parasitic world unlocks the secrets to its weakness.

Finally, the cost-effectiveness and accessibility of new anthelmintics are crucial considerations. Developing affordable drugs that are accessible to veterinarians and pet owners worldwide is essential for ensuring the widespread adoption of effective parasite control strategies. Equitable access to innovative therapeutics is paramount for global animal health. Cost-effectiveness must not come at the expense of quality or efficacy.

The challenge of anthelmintic resistance is multifaceted, requiring a multi-faceted solution. It requires a strategic investment in research and development, strong industry partnerships, and global cooperation to provide effective and accessible treatments. The welfare of companion animals depends on our ability to rise to this challenge. We must work together to secure a healthier future for our beloved pets. The future of veterinary parasitology hinges on our commitment to innovation and collaboration.

7.3 Research Directions

The fight against parasitic infections in companion animals demands continuous innovation. Future research should prioritize the development of novel anthelmintics with unique mechanisms of action, circumventing the resistance mechanisms prevalent in currently used drugs. This necessitates a deeper understanding of parasite genetics and molecular biology, enabling the identification of new drug targets. High-throughput screening methods, combined with advanced computational modeling, can accelerate the drug discovery process, identifying potential lead compounds that warrant further investigation. Furthermore, research into the development of parasite-specific vaccines holds immense promise. These vaccines could elicit protective immune responses, preventing infection or reducing parasite burdens, thus minimizing the reliance on chemical anthelmintics. This requires identification of appropriate immunogenic parasite antigens and development of effective vaccine delivery systems.

Investigating the complex interplay between parasite genetics, host immunity, and environmental factors is crucial. This holistic approach will enable the development of more effective and sustainable parasite control strategies. The use of "omics" technologies, such as genomics, transcriptomics, and proteomics, offers powerful tools to unravel these intricate interactions. Comparative studies across different parasite species and host breeds can pinpoint critical factors influencing parasite virulence and host susceptibility. By integrating these "omics" datasets with epidemiological data, we can refine our understanding of parasite transmission dynamics and identify high-risk populations.

Research into the development of diagnostic tools that are both rapid and cost-effective is also paramount. Point-of-care diagnostics would enable immediate diagnosis in veterinary clinics, facilitating timely and targeted treatment. This includes exploring the potential of advanced imaging techniques, such as advanced microscopy and spectroscopy, for rapid and non-invasive detection of parasites. Moreover, the development of improved diagnostic methods for detecting and quantifying anthelmintic resistance is critical for guiding treatment decisions and preventing the further spread of resistance. This will allow veterinarians to tailor treatment strategies based on accurate resistance profiles, minimizing the use of ineffective drugs and preserving the efficacy of existing anthelmintics.

A critical area of research is the investigation of environmentally friendly and sustainable parasite control strategies. This should include evaluating the efficacy and safety of botanical pesticides and other natural products, coupled with an extensive risk assessment of their potential impacts on the environment and animal health.

Furthermore, research into the development of integrated pest management (IPM) programs for companion animal parasites is essential. These programs should incorporate multiple strategies, such as environmental modification, sanitation, and behavioural changes, alongside targeted treatments. A comparative evaluation of the effectiveness and cost-efficiency of different IPM strategies is crucial for promoting the widespread adoption of sustainable parasite control practices.

Finally, understanding the zoonotic potential of parasitic infections is vital. Research into the transmission dynamics of zoonotic parasites, particularly those that can infect both companion animals and humans, is crucial for developing effective strategies to prevent human exposure. This includes the identification of high-risk populations and environments, the development of early warning systems for emerging zoonotic parasites, and the promotion of effective preventative measures for both humans and animals. Collaboration between veterinary parasitologists, human infectious disease specialists, and public health officials is crucial to address this shared challenge. This interdisciplinary approach can lead to more comprehensive parasite management strategies that address both animal and human health concerns, creating a one health approach to the field. Only through continuous research and innovation can we ensure the long-term health and well-being of companion animals in the face of evolving parasite threats.

7.4 Zoonotic Implications

The potential for zoonotic transmission—the spread of parasites from animals to humans—presents a significant public health concern. Many parasites infecting companion animals can also infect people, sometimes causing serious illness. Understanding these risks is crucial for both veterinary professionals and pet owners. Ignoring this aspect of parasite control is negligent and potentially dangerous. Effective parasite management in companion animals directly contributes to the safety of human populations, particularly children and immunocompromised individuals.

Effective control measures in veterinary practice are not just about animal health; they are about protecting the health of the human-animal bond and the wider community. This underscores the importance of preventive strategies, including regular parasite screening and appropriate treatment.

Think of Toxoplasma gondii, a parasite commonly found in cats. While usually asymptomatic in healthy adults, toxoplasmosis can pose severe risks during pregnancy, potentially leading to fetal abnormalities. Similarly, Echinococcus species, tapeworms found in dogs and foxes, can cause hydatid disease in humans, a potentially fatal condition if left untreated. These are not rare, isolated incidents; these are real-world dangers.

Therefore, implementing rigorous hygiene practices is paramount. This includes proper fecal waste disposal, thorough hand washing after handling pets, and minimizing direct contact with potentially contaminated environments. It's not simply enough to treat the animal; you must also protect the environment and the people around the animals.

Beyond the well-known examples, numerous other parasites pose a zoonotic threat. Several species of ticks can transmit Lyme disease and other bacterial infections, directly affecting human health. Fleas can carry diseases such as murine typhus, further highlighting the interconnectedness of animal and human health. This interconnectedness requires a unified approach to parasite control, with both veterinary and public health sectors working collaboratively.

This collaborative approach should include educational initiatives targeting pet owners, emphasizing responsible pet ownership and preventative strategies. Pet owners should be informed about the risks of zoonotic parasites and the importance of regular veterinary checkups, including parasite screenings. Clear, concise communication is essential, ensuring that owners can understand and implement the necessary preventative measures.

Furthermore, the role of public health agencies in surveillance and risk assessment cannot be overstated. Monitoring the prevalence of zoonotic parasites in animal populations and detecting outbreaks early are essential steps in protecting human health. This requires robust collaboration and data-sharing between veterinary and public health professionals. This exchange of vital information allows for a rapid and targeted response to emerging zoonotic threats.

Regular professional development and training for veterinarians and veterinary technicians are also critical. Staying updated on the latest advances in diagnostics, treatment protocols, and the emerging trends in zoonotic parasitology is an ongoing responsibility. This continuing education ensures that professionals are equipped to effectively manage both animal and public health risks. A proactive approach, both on an individual and a systemic level, is the key to effective zoonotic disease prevention.

The economic implications of zoonotic diseases must also be considered. Outbreaks can have significant effects on healthcare systems, requiring extensive resources for diagnosis, treatment, and public health interventions. Proactive measures in veterinary parasitology can significantly reduce this economic burden, ensuring the cost-effectiveness of parasite control strategies. It's a matter of public health and economics; prevention is far cheaper and more effective than treatment. In conclusion, the zoonotic implications of companion animal parasitism extend far beyond the individual animal. Comprehensive parasite control programs, incorporating preventative measures, early diagnosis, effective treatment, public health surveillance, and targeted education, are essential for protecting both animal and human health. A strong emphasis on prevention and a collaborative effort between veterinary professionals, pet owners, and public health agencies are vital in minimizing the risk and impact of zoonotic parasitic diseases. The health of our companion animals is intrinsically linked to our own; let us protect both.

7.5 Future Challenges

The rise of antimicrobial resistance presents a formidable challenge. Anthelmintics, while crucial in parasite control, are increasingly rendered ineffective by evolving parasite populations. This necessitates a multi-pronged approach, shifting from solely relying on chemical interventions to embracing integrated pest management strategies that minimize the selective pressure driving resistance. A concerted effort towards responsible drug use, including strict adherence to treatment protocols and strategic rotation of anthelmintics, is paramount. Furthermore, the development and implementation of novel diagnostic tools capable of rapidly identifying resistant strains will be essential for guiding targeted treatment decisions and limiting the spread of resistance. Failing to adapt our approaches will lead to treatment failures, prolonged suffering in animals, and increased veterinary costs. The consequences will be significant and far-reaching.

Research into alternative parasite control methods is vital. Exploring naturally derived compounds with anthelmintic properties, such as botanical extracts, offers a promising avenue for expanding our therapeutic arsenal. These natural alternatives could offer a reduced risk of resistance development compared to synthetic drugs. However, thorough investigation into their efficacy, safety, and potential side effects is crucial before widespread application. Equally important is the development of improved vaccines that target key parasite antigens. While the challenge of achieving broad-spectrum vaccine efficacy remains significant, focused research on specific parasitic diseases prevalent in certain geographic regions holds substantial promise.

Data collection and epidemiological surveillance play a crucial role. A robust data-gathering system that tracks parasite prevalence, resistance patterns, and treatment outcomes is essential. This information informs the development of evidence-based parasite control strategies, enabling veterinarians to make informed decisions about treatment choices and preventative measures. Such a system requires collaboration between veterinary practitioners, researchers, and public health agencies to ensure comprehensive data collection and timely dissemination of findings. Without this essential aspect, any effort towards controlling parasites will lack a crucial foundation of understanding.

The issue of zoonotic parasites necessitates heightened vigilance. Parasites capable of infecting both animals and humans pose a significant public health risk. Effective parasite control in companion animals indirectly contributes to human health protection. Therefore, greater collaboration between veterinary and human medicine is needed to monitor and manage these zoonotic threats. Public health awareness campaigns can help educate pet owners about the risks and promote responsible pet ownership practices that limit the transmission of these parasites to humans. Early detection and swift treatment, in both animals and humans, are essential in containing outbreaks and reducing the burden of disease.

Climate change is profoundly impacting parasite distribution and prevalence. Shifting temperature patterns and altered precipitation can expand the geographic range of certain parasites, increasing the risk of infection in previously unaffected areas. Understanding how climate change is influencing parasite ecology is vital for predicting future threats and adapting control strategies. Veterinary practitioners must stay updated on these changes to better anticipate and manage the potential spread of parasites in their specific regions. Preparation for these shifts will minimize disruptions in preventative and control methods.

The economic burden of parasitic diseases is substantial. The cost of diagnosis, treatment, and preventative measures adds up significantly for both pet owners and veterinary healthcare systems. Developing cost-effective parasite control strategies is paramount. This includes researching affordable yet effective diagnostic tools and anthelmintic alternatives, as well as promoting responsible pet ownership practices to minimize the risk of infection. Educating pet owners about the importance of preventive care, such as regular deworming and parasite preventative medications, can significantly reduce the overall economic burden associated with parasitic infections. The investment in research and preventive care will ultimately lead to more sustainable cost-effective parasite control.

www.ingramcontent.com/pod-product-compliance
Lightning Source LLC
LaVergne TN
LVHW022021200926
848481LV00007B/2465
9798348595654